FROM FLAB TO FAB

A guide to extreme fitness at home

No equipment needed!!! Just motivation!!!

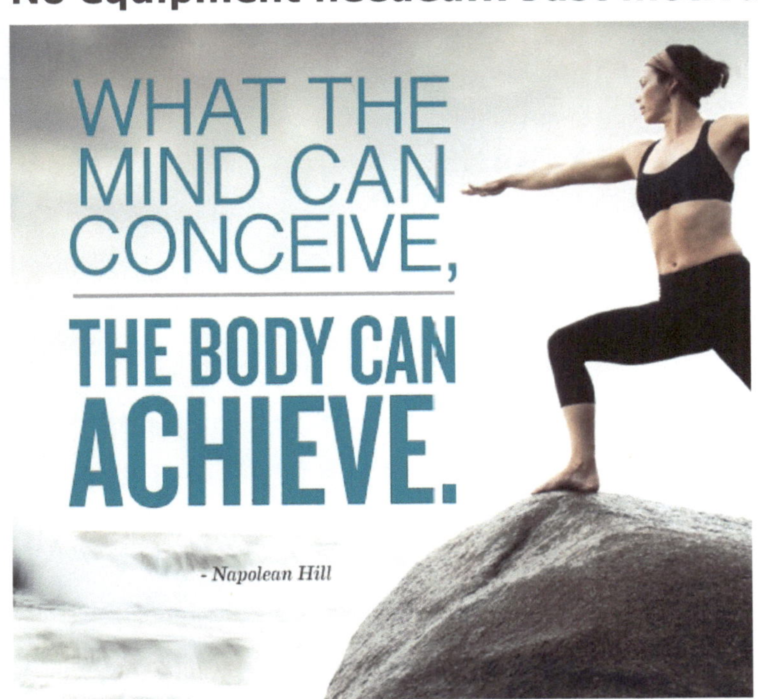

Shashank Singh Rathore

TABLE OF **CONTENTS**

WORK OUT SCHEDULE (XTREME)

Monthly Schedule						
Sun	Mon	Tue	Wed	Thu	Fri	Sat
	1 Tabata X	2 Chest, Back and Glutes X	3 10 * 10 X	4 Legs + Abs X	5 Cardio X	6 Yoga X
7 Rest/ Stretching	8 Arms X	9 Circuit X	10 Body Pump	11 Plyometric X	12 Running + Sprints X	13 Hiking/ Swimming/ Sports
14 Rest/ Stretching	15 Tabata X	16 Chest, Back and Glutes X	17 10 * 10 X	18 Legs + Abs X	19 Cardio X	20 Yoga
21 Rest/ Stretching	22 Arms X	23 Circuit X	24 Body Pump	25 Plyometric X	26 Running + Sprints X	27 Rock climb/ Sports/ combat
28 Rest/ Stretching	29 Tabata X	30 Chest, Back and Glutes X	31 10 * 10 X			

TABATA XTREME

A 60 min. workout for extreme drenching

- 4 rounds of 4 circuits
- Complete all circuits of Round 1 to 3, with 1 min. break between each circuit; and 3 min. break between each round
- Complete round 4 without any break
- Equipment needed
  - Water bottle
  - Towel
  - Yoga Mat (not necessary)

Dynamic Stretching – 5 min.

Warm Up – 5 min

- Jumping Jacks – 100
- High Knees – 100
- Mountain Climbers – 50
- Squats – 20
- Push Ups – 20

Tabata

Rounds	Exercise Time	Rest time in a circuit	Gap between 2 circuits	Rest after Round	Total Time
Round 1	20 sec	10 sec	1 min	3 min	14 min
Round 2	25 sec	5 sec	1 min	3 min	14 min
Round 3	30 sec	No rest	1 min	3 min	14 min
Round 4	15 sec	No rest	No rest	3 min	4 min

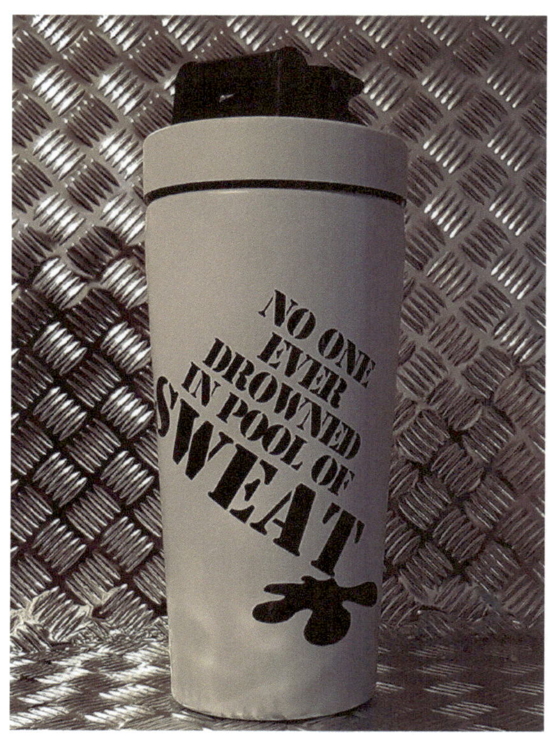

Circuits in each Round

- *Circuit 1 (Cardio)*

    o *Burpees + Push Ups*
    o *Mountain Climbers*
    o *High Knees*
    o *Double leg Mountain Climber*

- *Circuit 2 (Strength)*

    o *Push Ups*
    o *Squat Holds*
    o *Triceps Push Ups / Chair Dips*
    o *Alternate Lunges*

- ***Circuit 3 (Plyometrics)***

    o *Box Jumps*
    o *Skaters*
    o *Squat Thrusters + Push Ups*
    o *Squat Jumps*

- ***Circuit 4 (Core)***

    o *Plank Holds*
    o *Plan Jacks / Plank Ups*
    o *Russian Twists*
    o *Flutter Kicks*

Cool Down – 5 min.

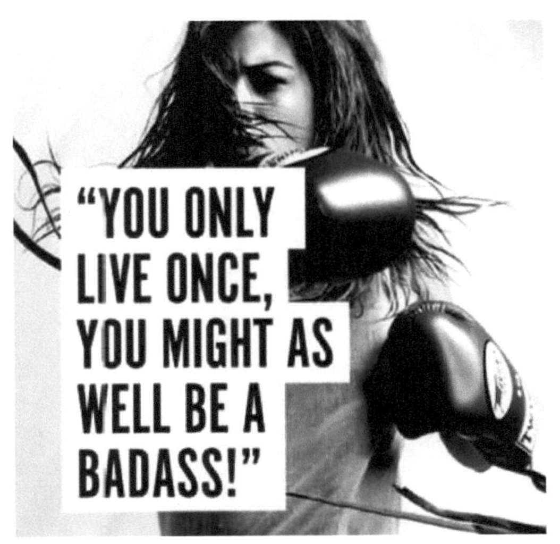

CHEST, BACK & GLUTES XTREME

A 60 min. workout for strengthening of chest, back and glute muscles

- 3 rounds of exercises for Chest, Back and Glutes
- Equipment needed
    - Water bottle and
    - Towel
    - Yoga Mat
    - Chair
    - Pull Up Bar
    - Resistance Band

Dynamic Stretching – 5 min.

Warm Up – 5 min

- 1 min jogging
- 1 min side to side (30 sec. each side)
- 30 sec frog walk
- 30 sec back run
- 30 sec lunge walk
- 30 sec jumping jacks
- 30 sec high knees
- 30 sec mountain climbers

* ***Back***

Exercise	Round 1	Round 2	Round 3
Overhead Pull Ups	Max.	Max.	Max.
Superman + Locust	10 + 10 sec. hold	10 + 10 sec. hold	10 + 10 sec. hold
Bird Dog + Flying Passe	10 (5 each side)	10 (5 each side)	10 (5 each side)
Reverse Snow Angels	10	10	10
Shoulder Bridge Up-down with single leg	20 (10 each leg)	20 (10 each leg)	20 (10 each leg)
Chin Ups	Max.	Max.	Max.
Twisters	20	20	20
Leg Up & Arm Pull	20 (10 each leg)	20 (10 each leg)	20 (10 each leg)

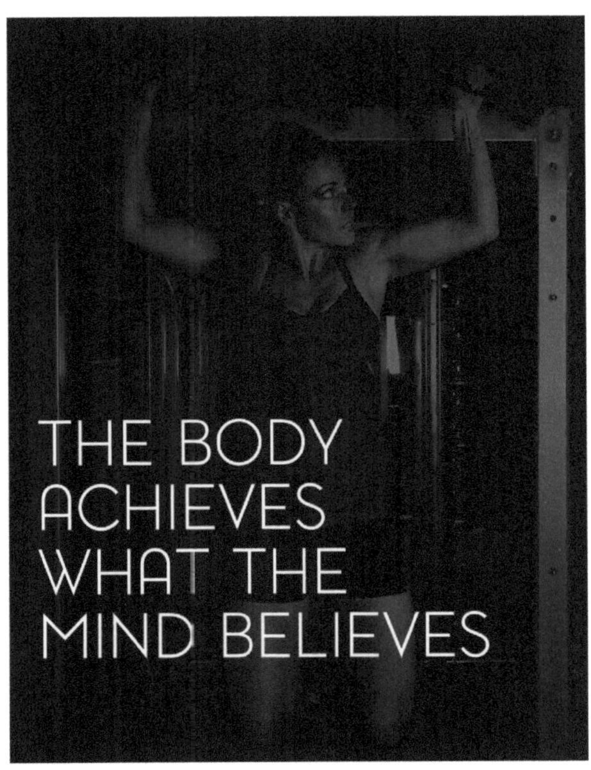

- ***Chest***

Exercise	Round 1	Round 2	Round 3
Push Ups	20	15	Max.
Push Up Hold	10 sec	10 sec	10 sec
Wide Hand Push Ups	15	12	Max.
Diamond Push Ups	12	10	Max.
Gorilla Push Ups/ Spiderman Push Ups	12	10	Max.
Decline Push Ups	12	10	Max.

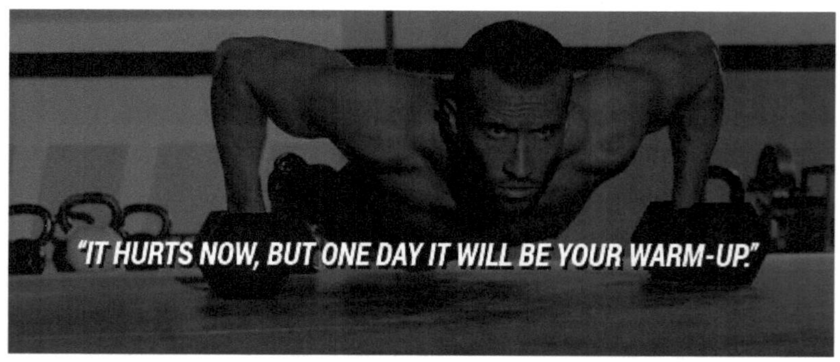

- ***Glutes***

Exercise	Round 1	Round 2	Round 3
Single leg squat	16 (8 each leg)	16 (8 each leg)	16 (8 each leg)
Fire Hydrant	20 (10 each leg)	20 (10 each leg)	20 (10 each leg)
Donkey kicks	20 (10 each leg)	20 (10 each leg)	20 (10 each leg)
V sit kick combo	20 (10 each leg)	20 (10 each leg)	20 (10 each leg)
Kick Back with resistance band	20 (10 each leg)	20 (10 each leg)	20 (10 each leg)
Side to side with resistance band	4 steps right and 4 steps left; repeat 5 times	4 steps right and 4 steps left; repeat 5 times	4 steps right and 4 steps left; repeat 5 times

Cool Down

10 * 10 XTREME

A 60 min. high intensity workout for endurance and fat loss

- 3 rounds of 10 exercises
- Only 10 repetition of 10 exercises per round; challenge is no rest between exercises
- 3 min. rest between each round
- Equipment needed
  - Water bottle
  - Towel
  - Yoga Mat (not necessary)

Dynamic Stretching – 5 min.

Warm Up – 5 min

- Jumping Jacks – 100
- High Knees – 100
- Mountain Climbers – 50
- Squats – 20
- Push Ups – 20

10 X 10 Xtreme workout

	Round 1	Round 2	Round 3
Burpees + Push Ups	10	10	10
Box Jump	10	10	10
Inch Warm + Push Ups	10	10	10
Jump Squats	10	10	10
Plank Ups	10	10	10
Squat Thrusters + Push Ups	10	10	10
Jump Lunges	20 (10 each leg)	20 (10 each leg)	20 (10 each leg)

Plank Jacks (10) + Double Leg Mountain Climbers (10)	10 + 10	10 + 10	10 + 10
Bird Dog + Flying Passe	10 (5 each leg)	10 (5 each leg)	10 (5 each leg)
Russian Twist (20) + Flutter Kicks (20)	20 (10 each leg) + 20 (10 each leg)	20 (10 each leg) + 20 (10 each leg)	20 (10 each leg) + 20 (10 each leg)

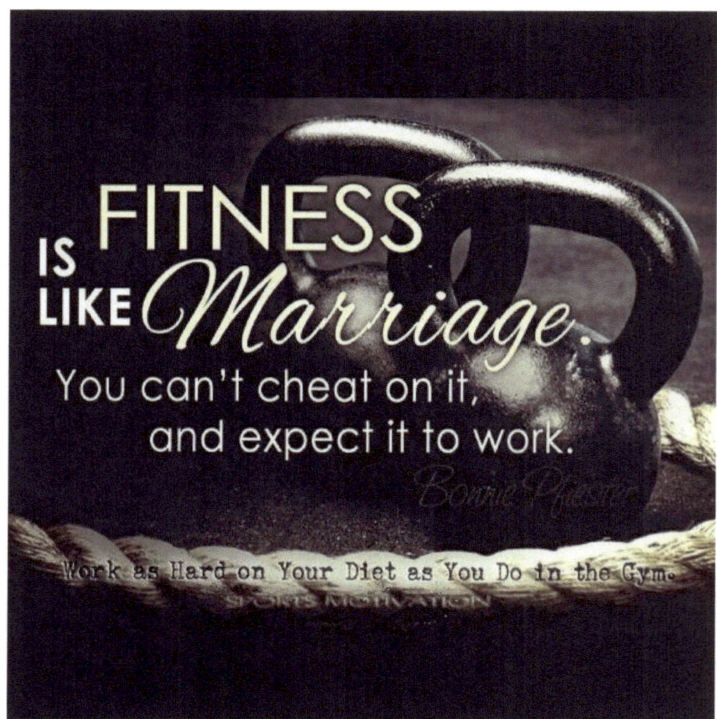

Cool Down

LEGS AND ABS XTREME

A 60 min. workout for strengthening of leg muscles and abs

- 3 rounds of exercises for Chest, Back and Glutes
- Equipment needed
  - Water bottle
  - Towel
  - Yoga Mat
  - Resistance Band

Dynamic Stretching – 5 min.

Warm Up – 6 min

- 1 min jogging
- 1 min side to side (30 sec. each side)
- 30 sec frog walk
- 30 sec back run
- 30 sec lunge walk
- 30 sec jumping jacks
- 30 sec high knees
- 30 sec mountain climbers
- 30 sec. double leg mountain climbers
- 30 sec. frog plank jumps

Strength Exercises

- *Legs*

Exercise	Round 1	Round 2	Round 3
Squat + Squat holds	20 30 sec hold	20 30 sec hold	20 30 sec hold
Lunges	15 each leg	15 each leg	15 each leg
Lunge Walk	Walk for 1 min	Walk for 1 min	Walk for 1 min
Pistol Squats	15 each leg	12 each leg	10 each leg
Wall Squat Hold	30 sec	30 sec	30 sec
Side to side lunge	20 (10 each leg)	20 (10 each leg)	20 (10 each leg)
Kick Back	15 each leg	15 each leg	15 each leg
Calf Raise	15 leg straight 15 toe touch 15 heel touch	15 leg straight 15 toe touch 15 heel touch	15 leg straight 15 toe touch 15 heel touch

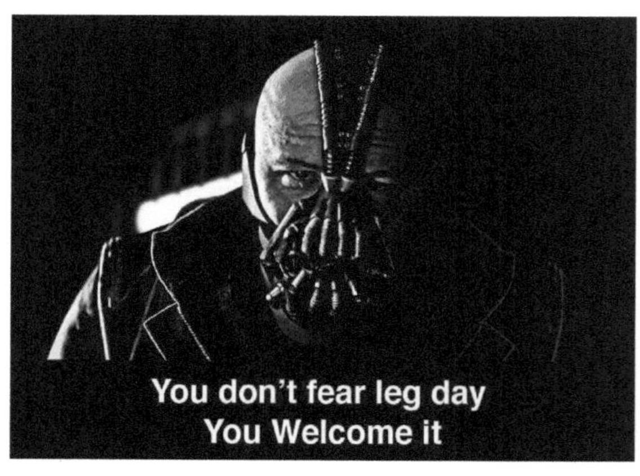

- *Abs*

Exercise	Round 1	Round 2	Round 3
Plank hold	30 sec hold	30 sec hold	30 sec hold
Plank Up	10	10	10
Plank Jacks	20	20	20
Sit Ups	15	15	15
Side to Side Sit Ups	20	20	20
Leg Up Sit Up	10	10	10
Russian Twist	20	20	20

Leg Raise (hold)	30 sec hold	30 sec hold	30 sec hold
Leg Raise (Up-Down)	15	15	15
Leg Raise (Fold and extend)	15	15	15
Leg Cycle	20	20	20
Flutter Kicks	20	20	20

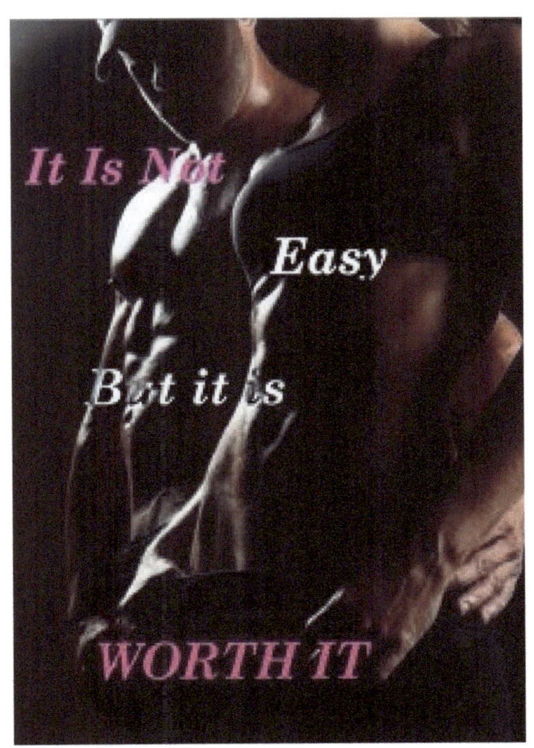

Cool Down

CARDIO XTREME

A 60 min. extreme cardio workout for weight loss and stamina improvement

- 4 circuits of cardio
- 2 rounds of each circuit
- 8 exercise in each circuit
- No break within a round, 1 min. break between 2 rounds
- 2 min. break between 2 circuits
- Equipment needed
  - Water bottle
  - Towel
  - Yoga Mat (not necessary)

Warm Up – 7 min

- 30 sec jogging
- 30 sec side to side (15 sec. each side alternate)
- 30 sec frog walk
- 30 sec lunge walk
- Jumping Jacks – 50
- High Knees – 50
- Mountain Climbers – 50
- Double leg mountain climbers – 25
- Frog plank jumps – 25
- Burpees – 5
- Squats – 20
- Push Ups – 10

Dynamic Stretching – 5 min.

Work-Out

- ***Circuit 1 (12 min.)***

Exercise	Round 1	1 min. break	Round 2
Sprints	30 sec		30 sec
Jumping Jacks	30 sec		30 sec
Burpees + Push Ups	30 sec		30 sec
Shadow Boxing	30 sec		30 sec
High Knees	30 sec		30 sec
Mountain Climbers	30 sec		30 sec
Side to Side Jumps	30 sec		30 sec
Squats	30 sec		30 sec

   - *2 min. break*

- ***Circuit 2 (12 min.)***

Exercise	Round 1	1 min. break	Round 2
Fast Squat Walk with hands on head	30 sec		30 sec
Star Jumps	30 sec		30 sec
Push Ups	30 sec		30 sec
Shadow Kick Boxing	30 sec		30 sec
Butt Kicks	30 sec		30 sec
Double legged Mountain Climbers	30 sec		30 sec
Skaters	30 sec		30 sec
Alt. Lunge Jumps	30 sec		30 sec

   - *2 min. break*

- *Circuit 3 (12 min.)*

Exercise	Round 1	1 min. break	Round 2
Sprints with side to side cone	30 sec		30 sec
Jump Squats	30 sec		30 sec
Inch Warm + Push Ups	30 sec		30 sec
Leg movements with guards up (Shadow Boxing)	30 sec		30 sec
Box/Tuck Jumps	30 sec		30 sec
Plank Jacks	30 sec		30 sec
Airborne Heisman	30 sec		30 sec
Lunge Walk	30 sec		30 sec

  o *2 min. break*

- *Circuit 4 (12 min.)*

Exercise	Round 1	1 min. break	Round 2
Sprints with touching floor by alt. hands	30 sec		30 sec
Oblique Jumping Jacks	30 sec		30 sec
Side Burpees (Side to side plank jump)	30 sec		30 sec
Front Back Jacks with side turns	30 sec		30 sec
Alt. Long Jumps	30 sec		30 sec
Frog Plank Jumps	30 sec		30 sec
Ski Jumps	30 sec		30 sec
Plank hold	30 sec		30 sec

  o *2 min. break*

Cool Down

YOGA XTREME

A 60 min. workout to relax and rejuvenate the body, improve posture and flexibility, and relieve mental stress and anxiety

- 10 series of 5 min. exercises for all body joints and muscles
- Equipment needed
    - Water bottle
    - Towel
    - Yoga Mat

Series 1 – Pranayama (Breathing for lungs & blood circulation) – 10 min.

- *Breathe Retention*
    - *Sit into Padmasana pose (leg crossed)*
    - *Take a deep breathe slowly*
    - *Hold for 10 sec*
    - *Breathe out till max slowly*
    - *Repeat 10 times*
- *Kapal Bhati*
    - *Sit into Padmasana pose (leg crossed)*
    - *Take a deep breathe*
    - *Breathe out fast and tighten stomach*
    - *Repeat 25 times*
- *Lion Pose*
    - *Sit into Padmasana pose (leg crossed)*
    - *Take a deep breathe*
    - *Breathe out fast from mouthe and tighten stomach*
    - *Repeat 25 times*
- *Nadi Shodhana*
    - *Sit into Padmasana pose (leg crossed)*
    - *Close left nostril*
    - *Take a deep breath slowly from right nostril*

- o *Close right nostril and breathe out from left nostril*
- o *Breathe in from left nostril, close left nostril and breathe out from right nostril*
- o *Repeat 10 times*

Warm Up – 5 min

- *Neck Stretch*
- *Arm Stretch*
- *Triceps and Biceps Stretch*
- *Wrist Stretch*
- *Back Stretch*
- *Forward and backward bend*
- *Lunge Stretch*
- *Hamstring Stretch*
- *Toe Stretch*

Series 2 – Sun Salutations (Full Body condition) – 15 min

- Sun Salutation
    - o *(inhale) Mountain pose*
    - o *(exhale) standing forward bend*
    - o *(inhale) half standing forward bend*
    - o *(exhale) low plank/chaturanga*
    - o *(inhale) upward facing dog*
    - o *(exhale) downward facing dog*
    - o *(inhale) Move alternate (right/left) leg forward to runners pose*
    - o *(exhale) Move other leg forward to standing forward bend*
    - o *(inhale) Mountain pose*
    - o *(exhale) Namaste pose*
    - o *Repeat 6 times*

- Warrior 1, Warrior 2 and Reverse Warrior
  - *(inhale) Mountain pose*
  - *(exhale) standing forward bend*
  - *(inhale) half standing forward bend*
  - *(exhale) low plank/chaturanga*
  - *(inhale) upward facing dog*
  - *(exhale) downward facing dog*
  - *(inhale) Move right leg forward to runners pose*
  - *(exhale) Move to Warrior 1 pose*
  - *(inhale) Move to Warrior 2 pose*
  - *(exhale) Move to Reverse Warrior pose*
  - *(inhale) Move to Warrior 2 pose*
  - *(exhale) Move to Warrior 1 pose*
  - *(inhale) Move to runners pose*
  - *(exhale) Move to high plank pose*
  - *(exhale) low plank/chaturanga*
  - *(inhale) upward facing dog*
  - *(exhale) downward facing dog*
  - *(inhale) Move alternate (right/left) leg forward to runners pose*
  - *(exhale) Move other leg forward to standing forward bend*
  - *(inhale) Mountain pose*
  - *(exhale) Namaste pose*
  - *Repeat 4 times*

- Warrior 3, Half Moon and Triangle Pose
  - *(inhale) Mountain pose*
  - *(exhale) standing forward bend*
  - *(inhale) half standing forward bend*
  - *(exhale) low plank/chaturanga*
  - *(inhale) upward facing dog*
  - *(exhale) downward facing dog*
  - *(inhale) Move right leg forward to runners pose*
  - *(exhale) Move to Warrior 1 pose*

- o *(inhale) Move to Warrior 2 pose*
  - o *(exhale) Move to Warrior 3 pose*
  - o *(inhale) Move to Half Moon pose*
  - o *(exhale) Move to Warrior 3 pose*
  - o *(inhale) Move to Warrior 2 pose*
  - o *(exhale) Move to triangle pose*
  - o *(inhale) Move to single leg forward bend (hamstring stretch)*
  - o *(exhale) Move to reverse triangle*
  - o *(inhale) Move to single leg forward bend*
  - o *(exhale) Move to lunge pose*
  - o *(inhale) Move to Warrior 2 pose*
  - o *(exhale) Move to Warrior 1 pose*
  - o *(inhale) Move to runners pose*
  - o *(exhale) Move to high plank pose*
  - o *(exhale) low plank/chaturanga*
  - o *(inhale) upward facing dog*
  - o *(exhale) downward facing dog*
  - o *(inhale) Move alternate (right/left) leg forward to runners pose*
  - o *(exhale) Move other leg forward to standing forward bend*
  - o *(inhale) Mountain pose*
  - o *(exhale) Namaste pose*
  - o *Repeat 4 times*

- Chair Pose
  - o *(inhale) Mountain pose*
  - o *(exhale) standing forward bend*
  - o *(inhale) half standing forward bend*
  - o *(exhale) low plank/chaturanga*
  - o *(inhale) upward facing dog*
  - o *(exhale) downward facing dog*
  - o *(inhale) Jump to half standing forward bend*
  - o *(exhale) Move to Chair Pose*

- o *(inhale) Move to Mountain pose*
- o *(exhale) Move to twisted Chair Pose*
- o *(inhale) Move to Mountain pose*
- o *(exhale) Move to twisted Chair Pose (other side)*
- o *(inhale) Mountain pose*
- o *(exhale) Namaste pose*
- o *Repeat 2 times*

Series 3 – Standing Stretch (improve flexibility) – 15 min

- Tree
  - o *(inhale) Fold 1 leg with its heel placed on quadriceps of other; stand on other leg and into Namaste pose*
  - o *(exhale) Move to mountain pose on 1 leg*
  - o *(inhale) Move to Namaste pose with the leg folded and heels places on quadriceps of other*
  - o *(exhale) Move into standing pose*
  - o *Repeat 2 times with each leg*

- Royal Dancer Stretch
  - o *(inhale) Fold 1 leg and move to quadriceps stretch*
  - o *(exhale) Stretch opposite hand and folded leg to move to Royal Dancer pose*
  - o *(inhale) Move to quadriceps stretch*
  - o *(exhale) Move into standing pose*
  - o *Repeat 2 times with each leg*

- Standing Leg Extension
  - o *(inhale) Fold 1 leg into high knee pose*
  - o *(exhale) Straighten the leg and lock the toe with same hand*
  - o *(inhale) Move back to high knee pose*
  - o *(exhale) Move into standing pose*
  - o *Repeat 2 times with each leg*
  - o 30 sec lunge walk

- Hamstring and Lunge Stretch
    - *(inhale) Spread the legs forward/backward and move into mountain pose*
    - *(exhale) With legs straight, move into Hamstring stretch*
    - *(inhale) Move into runners pose*
    - *(exhale) Move into lunge position*
    - *(inhale) Move into runners pose and then to move leg forward into bend knee pose*
    - *(exhale) Move into standing pose*
    - *Repeat 2 times with each leg*

- Garland Pose
    - *(inhale) Stand into Tadasana Pose*
    - *(exhale) Squat with your feet as close together as possible*
    - *(inhale) Separate your thighs slightly wider than your torso*
    - *(exhale) Lean your torso forward and fit it snugly between your thighs*
    - *(inhale) Press your elbows against your inner knees, bringing your palms, and resist the knees into the elbows. This will help lengthen your front torso*
    - *(exhale) Press your inner thighs against the sides of your torso. Reach your arms forward, then swing them out to the sides and notch your shins into your armpits. Press your finger tips to the floor, or reach around the outside of your ankles and clasp your back heels.*
    - *(inhale) Straighten legs into forward bend*
    - *(exhale) Move into Namaste pose*
    - *Repeat 2 times*

- Crow Pose
    - *(inhale) Stand into Tadasana Pose*

- o *(exhale) Squat down with your inner feet a few inches apart. Separate your knees wider than your hips and lean the torso forward, between the inner thighs. Stretch your arms forward, then bend your elbows, place your hands on the floor and the backs of the upper arms against the shins*
- o *(inhale) Snuggle your inner thighs against the sides of your torso, and your shins into your armpits, and slide the upper arms down as low onto the shins as possible. Lift up onto the balls of your feet and lean forward even more, taking the weight of your torso onto the backs of the upper arms. To help yourself do this, keep your tailbone as close to your heels as possible*
- o *(exhale) Lean forward even more onto the backs of your upper arms, to the point where the balls of your feet leave the floor. Now your torso and legs are balanced on the backs of your upper arms.*
- o *(inhale) Move back into squat position*
- o *(exhale) Move into Namaste pose*
- o *Repeat twice*

Series 4 – Seated Stretch (improves flexibility) – 15 min

- Seated Hamstring Stretch
  - o *Sit on both legs*
  - o *(inhale) Raise both hands and chest*
  - o *(exhale) Bend forward and hold. Try to move the back forward as much as possible*
  - o *Repeat 4 times*
  - o *Fold left leg and place feet on right side quadriceps*
  - o *(inhale) Raise both hands and chest*
  - o *(exhale) Bend forward towards right leg and hold. Try to move the back forward as much as possible*
  - o *Repeat with other leg*
  - o *Repeat twice*

- o *Fold left leg and place feet above right leg*
  - o *(inhale) Raise both hands and chest*
  - o *(exhale) Bend forward towards right leg and hold*
  - o *Repeat with other leg*
  - o *Repeat twice*
  - o *Straighten both legs and stretch them outwards*
  - o *(inhale) Raise both hands and chest*
  - o *(exhale) Bend forward towards right leg and hold*
  - o *(inhale) Raise both hands and chest*
  - o *(exhale) Bend forward towards left leg and hold*
  - o *(inhale) Raise both hands and chest*
  - o *(exhale) Bend forward and hold*
  - o *Repeat twice*

- **Butterfly Stretch**
  - o *Sit on both legs and join heels*
  - o *Lock both feet by hands*
  - o *Flap legs up-down 10 times*
  - o *Move legs down and hold*
  - o *Repeat twice*

- **Seated Spinal Stretch**
  - o *Sit on both legs*
  - o *Grab right ankle by right hand and put it under and behind left leg*
  - o *Grab left foot and put it over right leg*
  - o *(inhale) Straighten right hand and raise vertically and put left hand on spine behind*
  - o *(exhale) Twist back from left side*
  - o *(inhale) Move to previous position*
  - o *Repeat with other leg*
  - o *Repeat twice*

- **Seated Glute Stretch**

- o *Sit on both legs*
  - o *Put left foot behind and place left quadriceps on floor*
  - o *Fold right leg*
  - o *Take a deep breadth*
  - o *(exhale) Bend forward*
  - o *Repeat with other leg*
  - o *Repeat twice*

- Cat Stretch
  - o *Sit on both hands and legs*
  - o *(inhale) Head up and chest down*
  - o *(exhale) Head down and chest up*
  - o *Repeat 5 times*

- Cobra Stretch and Child's pose
  - o *Lie down on stomach*
  - o *(inhale) Move to cobra position*
  - o *(exhale) Move to child's pose*
  - o *Repeat twice*
  - o *(inhale) Move to cobra position*
  - o *(exhale) Lock back on right side and stretch*
  - o *Repeat other side*
  - o *Repeat twice*
  - o *(inhale) Move to cobra position*
  - o *(exhale) Move to child's pose*
  - o *Put both hands on right side and stretch*
  - o *Repeat on left side*

- Frog Stretch
  - o *Sit on both hands and legs*
  - o *Fold hands to plank*
  - o *Spread legs outwards and hold into frog pose*

- Ankle Stretch

- o *Sit on both heels on Bhajrasan pose and hold*
- o *Move legs outwards and hold*
- o *Lean back on the hands*
- o *After a few moments, bring the hands to the floor beside your legs and lean back as much as possible*

- **Bow Pose**
  - o *Lie on belly with hands alongside torso, palms up*
  - o *(inhale) Bend right knee and hold with right hand. Hold*
  - o *(exhale) Lift knee and hands with just stomach touching floor*
  - o *Repeat with other leg*
  - o *Repeat twice*
  - o *(exhale) Bend your knees, bringing your heels as close as you can to your buttocks. Reach back with your hands and take hold of your ankles (but not the tops of the feet).*
  - o *(inhale) Lift your heels away from your buttocks and, at the same time, lift your thighs away from the floor. This will have the effect of pulling your upper torso and head off the floor. Burrow the tailbone down toward the floor, and keep your back muscles soft. As you continue lifting the heels and thighs higher, press your shoulder blades firmly against your back to open your heart. Draw the tops of the shoulders away from your ears. Gaze forward.*
  - o *(exhale) Hold*
  - o *Repeat twice*

- **Table**
  - o *Sit on both legs*
  - o *Move to crab position*
  - o *Move to table and hold*
  - o *Repeat twice*

- Bridge
  - *Lie down on back. Make sure dist. Between toes and heels is same*
  - *Roll up on shoulders to bridge pose and hold*
  - *Relax*
  - *Move back to bridge*
  - *Turn hands back over the body and lift body on hands to make a complete bridge on hands and legs*
  - *Repeat twice*

- Lying Glute and Hamstring Stretch
  - *Lie down on back*
  - *Fold right leg and hold right calf with both hands*
  - *Turn folded right leg outwards with right hand and look on left side*
  - *Turn folded right leg inwards with left hand and look on right side*
  - *Repeat with other leg*
  - *Fold left leg and place on right quadriceps. Hold right calf by both hands and pull towards chest. Hold*
  - *Repeat with other leg*
  - *Fold both legs and lock calves by both hands. Pull towards chest.*
  - *Try to touch knees with face and hold*
  - *Roll back and forth 5 times*
  - *make a complete bridge on hands and legs*

- Shoulder Stand
  - *Lie down on back*
  - *Move to plough position and hold*
  - *Put hands on back and straighten legs in vertical direction*
  - *Move to shoulder stand*
  - *Repeat twice*

- Happy Baby
  - *Lie down on back*
  - *Bend legs and hold toes with hands*
  - *Twist right and left side 10 times*

- Child's Pose
  - *Sit on knees*
  - *Move forward to child's pose*
  - *Hold and relax*

- Shavasana (2 min.)
  - *Lie down on back*
  - *Relax to sleeping pose*
  - *Deep breath, hold and release observing breath 10 times*
  - *Deep breath thinking of all body parts and release negative energy via breath*

Series 5 – Meditation (5 min)

- *Meditation Pose*
  - *Sit down on both legs and fold legs into Padmasana pose*
  - *Take deep breath, hold and release*
  - *Think only of breath, nothing else*

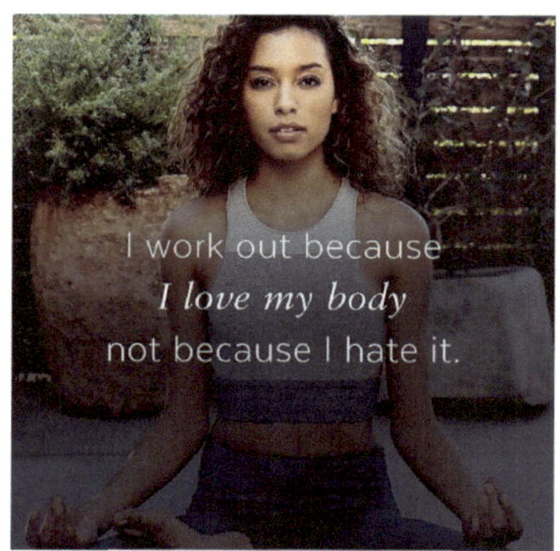

ARMS XTREME

A 60 min. workout for arms conditioning

- 3 rounds of exercises for Shoulders, Biceps and Triceps
- Equipment needed
  - Water bottle
  - Towel
  - Yoga Mat
  - Chair
  - Light Dumbbells
  - Medium weight Dumbbells

Dynamic Stretching – 5 min.

Warm Up – 6 min

- 1 min jogging
- 1 min side to side (30 sec. each side)
- 30 sec high knees
- 30 sec butt kicks
- 30 sec frog walk
- 30 sec crab walk
- 30 sec frog plank jumps
- 30 sec plank jacks
- 30 sec arm circles
- 30 sec inchworm

- *Shoulders*

Exercise	Round 1	Round 2	Round 3
Arm Circles clockwise (lower radius)	30 sec	30 sec	30 sec
Larm Circles anticlockwise (larger radius)	30 sec	30 sec	30 sec
Shoulder tap on plank	20	20	20
Inch worm	10	10	10
Shoulder Press (Medium wts.)	10	10	10
Upright Rows (Medium wts)	10	10	10
Arm Flys (Light wts.)	10	10	10

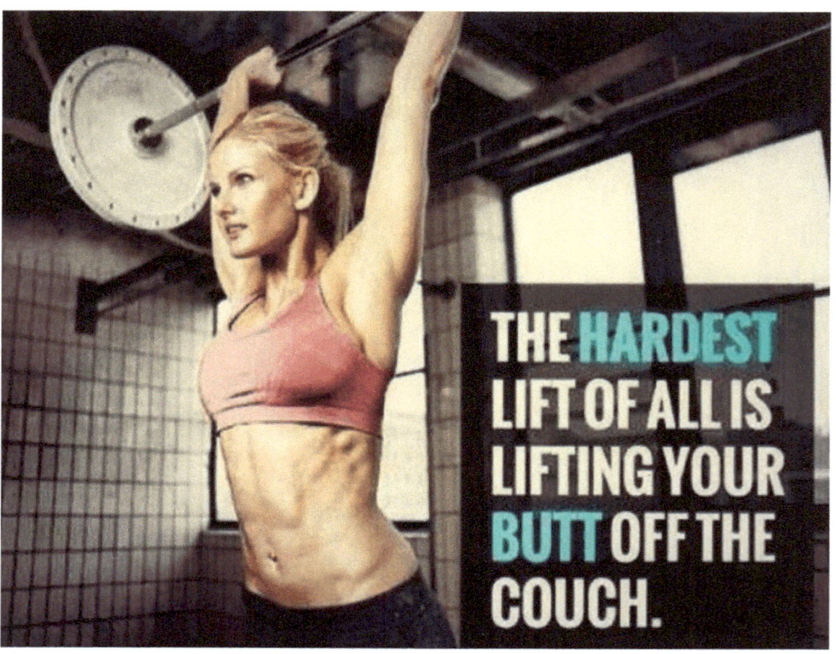

* ***Triceps***

Exercise	Round 1	Round 2	Round 3
Chair Dips	15	15	15
Triceps Push Ups	10	10	10
Triceps Extension Push Ups	10	10	10
Side Tri Rise	10 each side	10 each side	10 each side
Standing triceps extension (medium wts.)	15	15	15
Lying triceps extension (medium wts.)	10	10	10
Triceps Kick Back (Light wts.)	10 each side	10 each side	10 each side

* ***Biceps***

Exercise	Round 1	Round 2	Round 3
Pike Press	15	15	15
Crab Walk	30 sec	30 sec	30 sec
Side Plank Push Up + Rotation	10 each side alternating	10 each side alternating	10 each side alternating
Biceps Curls (medium wts.)	10	10	10
Straight – Out – In Biceps Curls (medium wts.)	5 each type	5 each type	5 each type
Hammer Curl (medium wts.)	10	10	10
Static Arm Curls (medium wts.)	4*4 alternating	4*4 alternating	4*4 alternating
Crouching Cohen Curls (medium wts.)	10	10	10

| 3 * 21 biceps curls (light weight) | 21 | 21 | 21 |

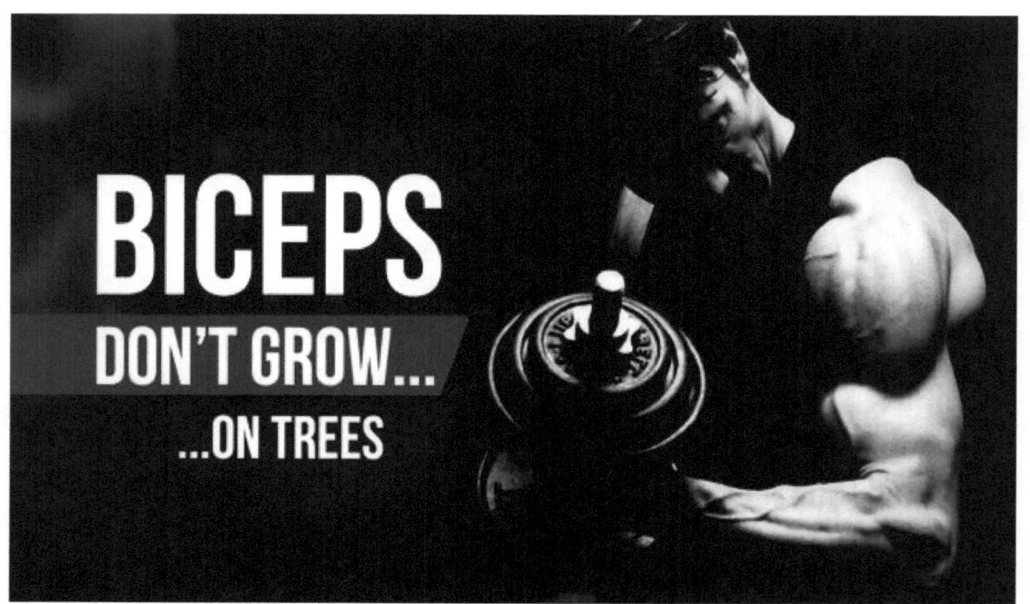

Cool Down

CIRCUIT XTREME

A 60 min. cross body workout with compound exercise to attain lean body

- 2 rounds of 5 circuits
- 2 exercise in each circuit
- 20 sec each excercise
- Round 1 for 2 min. and Round 2 for 3 min.
- 1 min break between 2 rounds
- 1 min break between 2 circuits
- Equipment needed
  - Water bottle
  - Towel
  - Stepper
  - Yoga Mat (not necessary)

Dynamic Stretching – 5 min.

Warm Up – 5 min

- Running – 1 min
- Frog Walk – 30 sec
- Lunge Walk – 30 sec
- Jumping Jacks – 100
- High Knees – 100
- Mountain Climbers – 50
- Squats – 20
- Push Ups – 20

Circuits	Round 1	Gap between 2 rounds	Round 2	Gap between 2 circuits	Total Time
Circuit 1	2 min	1 min	3 min	2 min	8 min
Circuit 2	2 min	1 min	3 min	2 min	8 min
Circuit 3	2 min	1 min	3 min	2 min	8 min
Circuit 4	2 min	1 min	3 min	2 min	8 min
Circuit 5	2 min	1 min	3 min	2 min	8 min

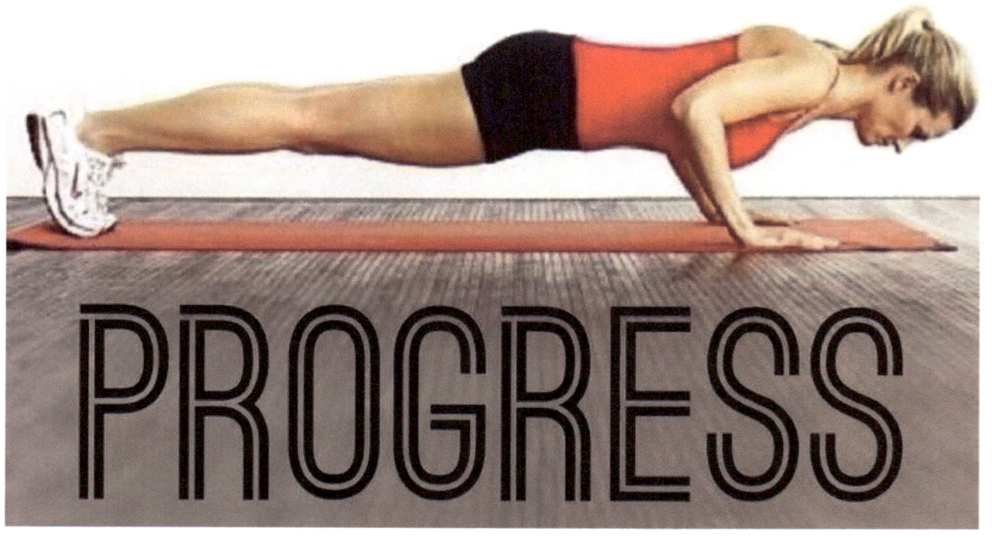

33

Circuits

- ***Circuit 1 (Cardio)***

    - *Stepper/Jumping Jack (20 sec)*
    - *High Knees (20 sec)*

- ***Circuit 2 (Upper Strength)***

    - *Burpees/Push Ups/Inchworm (20 sec)*
    - *Crab Walk/Dips/Pike Press (20 sec)*

- ***Circuit 3 (Plyometrics)***

    - *Box Jumps (20 sec)*
    - *Squat Jumps (20 sec)*

- ***Circuit 4 (Lower Strength)***

    - *Squat Holds (20 sec)*
    - *Lunge Walk (20 sec)*

- ***Circuit 4 (Core)***

    - *Plank Holds/Plank Ups (20 sec)*
    - *Flutter Kicks/Russian Twist (20 sec)*

Cool Down – 5 min.

BODY PUMP XTREME

A 60 min. workout for body conditioning and muscle definition

- Full body workout
- 6 circuits
- No break within a circuit
- 1 min rest between 2 circuits
- Equipment needed
    - Water bottle
    - Towel
    - 1 Stepper
    - 1 weight bar
    - Medium to light weights
    - Yoga Mat (not necessary)

Dynamic Stretching – 5 min.

Warm Up – 5 min

- Running – 1 min
- Jumping Jacks – 30 sec
- High Knees – 30 sec
- Squats – 20
- Lunges – 20
- Push Ups – 20
- Dead Lift – 20
- Shoulder Press – 20
- Biceps Curls – 20
- Triceps Extensions – 20

Body Pump Work-Out

- *Circuit 1 – Chest*

Exercise	Round 1	Round 2
Chest Press • *4 reps – 3 count* • *4 reps – 2 count* • *8 singles*	45 sec	45 sec
Push Ups • *4 reps – 3 count* • *4 reps – 2 count* • *8 singles*	45 sec	45 sec
Side Lateral Rise • *4 reps – 3 count* • *4 reps – 2 count* • *8 singles*	45 sec	45 sec

- *Circuit 2 – Legs*

Exercise	Round 1	Round 2
Squat into Shoulder Press • *4 reps – 3 count* • *4 reps – 2 count* • *8 singles*	45 sec	45 sec
Sumo Squat • *4 reps – 3 count* • *4 reps – 2 count* • *8 singles*	45 sec	45 sec
Low Squat Pulses	30 sec	30 sec

- *Circuit 3 – Back*

Exercise	Round 1	Round 2
Dead Lift • *4 reps – 3 count* • *4 reps – 2 count* • *8 singles*	60 sec	60 sec

Bent Over Row
    • *4 reps – 3 count*
    • *4 reps – 2 count*
    • *8 singles*		

Plank Row • *Singles – 10 each side*	45 sec	45 sec
Dead Lift into row • *10 singles*	45 sec	45 sec

- ***Circuit 4 – Biceps***

Exercise	Round 1	Round 2

Biceps Curl
    • *4 reps – 3 count*
    • *4 reps – 2 count*
    • *8 singles*
	45 sec	45 sec

Hammer Curl
    • *4 reps – 3 count*
    • *4 reps – 2 count*
    • *8 singles*
	45 sec	45 sec

Biceps Curl • *3 * 21*	30 sec	30 sec

- ***Circuit 5 – Triceps***

Exercise	Round 1	Round 2
Dips on stepper • *20 singles*	45 sec	45 sec

Triceps extension sitting on stepper
    • *4 reps – 3 count*
    • *4 reps – 2 count*
    • *8 singles*
	45 sec	45 sec

Incline Triceps Push Ups on stepper • *16 singles*	45 sec	45 sec

- *Circuit 6 – Glutes, Hips and Hamstrings*

Exercise	Round 1	Round 2
Weighted Static Lunge (Left) • *4 reps – 3 count* • *4 reps – 2 count* • *8 singles*	45 sec	45 sec
Weighted Static Lunge (Right) • *4 reps – 3 count* • *4 reps – 2 count* • *8 singles*	45 sec	45 sec
Glute Bridge • *Weight on stomach – 24* • *Left leg lifted – 24 reps* • *Right leg lifted – 24 reps*	45 sec	45 sec
Alternating Back Lunge with weight held in front • *8 reps each side*	30 sec	30 sec

- *Circuit 7 – Shoulders*

Exercise	Round 1	Round 2
Shoulder Press • *4 reps – 3 count* • *4 reps – 2 count* • *8 singles*	45 sec	45 sec
Upright Rows • *4 reps – 3 count* • *4 reps – 2 count* • *8 singles*	45 sec	45 sec
Arm Flys • *4 reps – 3 count* • *4 reps – 2 count* • *8 singles*	45 sec	45 sec

- *Circuit 8 – Core*

Exercise	Round 1	Round 2
Plank with arm taps • *8 reps each side*	20 sec	20 sec
Plank with toe taps • *8 reps each side*	20 sec	20 sec
3 crouch crunches – 8 reps	20 sec	20 sec
Crouch singles – 16 reps	20 sec	20 sec
Plank Hold	60 sec	60 sec
Leg lifts – 16 reps	20 sec	20 sec
Weighted crunch with 1 leg extended – 16	20 sec	20 sec

Cool Down – 5 min.

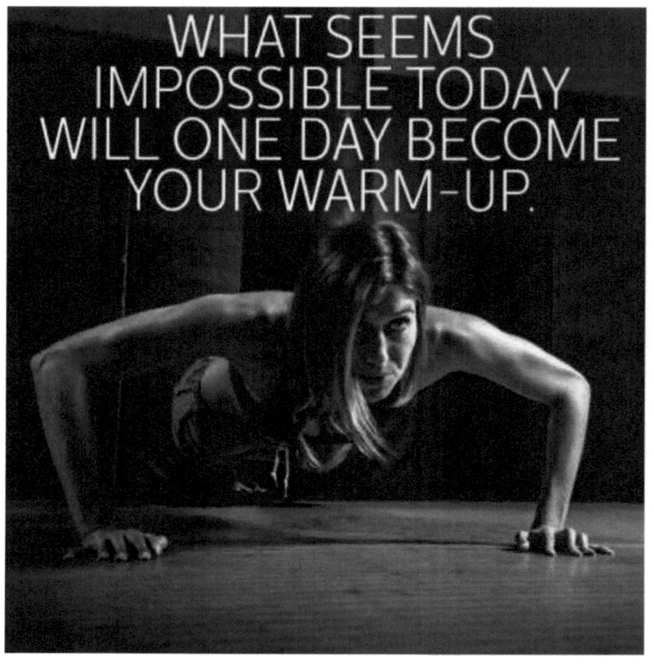

PYLOMETRICS XTREME

A 60 min. high plyometrics workout for endurance and fat loss

- 6 circuits with 2 rounds each
- Every round is for 2 min. (No rest)
- 1 min. rest between rounds
- 2 min. rest between 2 circuits
- Equipment needed
  - Water bottle
  - Towel
  - Yoga Mat (not necessary)

Dynamic Stretching – 5 min.

Warm Up – 5 min

- Jumping Jacks – 100
- High Knees – 100
- Mountain Climbers – 50
- Squats – 20
- Push Ups – 20

Plyometrics Work-Out

- ***Circuit 1 (7 min.)***

Exercise	Round 1	1 min. break	Round 2
Jump Squats	30 sec		30 sec
Run Stance Squats	30 sec		30 sec
Airborne Heisman	30 sec		30 sec
Swing Kicks	30 sec		30 sec

  - *2 min. break*

- ***Circuit 2 (7 min.)***

Exercise	Round 1	1 min. break	Round 2
Squat Reach Jump	30 sec		30 sec
Run Stance Squat Reach Pick Ups	30 sec		30 sec
Double Airborne Heisman	30 sec		30 sec
Circle Run	30 sec		30 sec

  - *2 min. break*

- ***Circuit 3 (7 min.)***

Exercise	Round 1	1 min. break	Round 2
Jump Knee Tucks	30 sec		30 sec
Mary Katherine Lunges	30 sec		30 sec
Leapfrog Squats	30 sec		30 sec
Twist Combos	30 sec		30 sec

  - *2 min. break*

- *Circuit 4 (7 min.)*

Exercise	Round 1	1 min. break	Round 2
Rock Star Hops	30 sec		30 sec
Gap Jumps	30 sec		30 sec
Squat Jacks	30 sec		30 sec
Military March	30 sec		30 sec

  - *2 min. break*

- *Circuit 5 (7 min.)*

Exercise	Round 1	1 min. break	Round 2
Run Squat 180 Jump Switch	30 sec		30 sec
Lateral Leapfrog Squats	30 sec		30 sec
Monster Truck Tire Jumps	30 sec		30 sec
Hot Foot	30 sec		30 sec

  - *2 min. break*

- *Circuit 6 (7 min.)*

Exercise	Round 1	1 min. break	Round 2
Pitch and Catch	30 sec		30 sec
Jump Shots	30 sec		30 sec
Football Hero	30 sec		30 sec
Sprints	30 sec		30 sec

  - *2 min. break*

Cool Down

RUNNING XTREME

Outdoor workout to transform your body from walking to running in 12 weeks

Week 1 (3 sets)

- *15 min running*
- *3 min rest*

Week 2 (2 sets)

- *20 min running*
- *3 min walk*
- *2 min rest*

Week 3 (3 sets)

- *10 min running*
- *1 min sprint*
- *4 min walk*

Week 4 (2 sets)

- *25 min running*
- *5 min walk*

Week 5 (5 sets)

- *9 min running*
- *1 min sprint*
- *2 min walk*

Week 6

- *40 min running*
- *5 min walk*
- *15 min running*

Week 7 (5 sets)

- *8 min running*
- *1 min sprint*
- *2 min walk*

Week 8 (2 sets)

- *28 min running*
- *1 min sprint*
- *1 min walk*

Week 9 (10 sets)

- *4 min running*
- *1 min sprint*
- *1 min walk*

Week 10

- *60 min running*
- *1 min sprint*

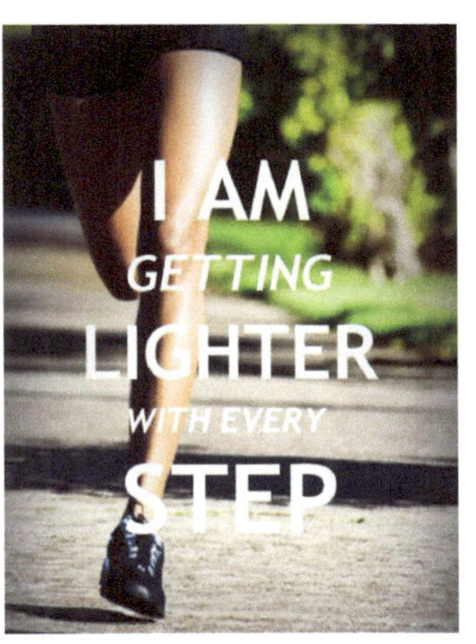